My Gratitude Journal

This journal belongs to _____

Reward: _____ scoops of ice cream

In this world, we may always want more
We already have much to be grateful for

Written by Simar Mangat
Cover Design by Avina Harry
www.wethehappyclub.com

Lion Rose Henna
Designs by Avina
LionRoseHenna On etsy.com

Intentions and Commitments

If you go through the exercises in this journal daily, you will almost definitely be a **happier, more grateful, and resilient** person. Before we embark, however, let's paint a picture of how you're going to go about this. When we consciously plan and set an intention for any activity, we're far more likely to get what we want from it.

Intentions

What would I like to get out of this gratitude journal?

_____

_____

What excites me most about gratitude journaling?

_____

_____

Committments

I plan to spend _____ (amount of time) journaling every _____ (day, week) in the _____(morn, night, etc.)

What challenges/obstacles may get in the way?

_____

_____

How will I respond to these challenges?

_____

_____

Your Journaling Guide

The Why:

Happiness is a skill, just like any other, you can master through **deliberate practice**. Gratitude journaling is one such practice that serves as the mental equivalent of getting in shape. I've personally found the journal to be incredibly grounding during my time at Stanford.

Turns out, some of the world's most successful people like **Oprah** also gratitude journal every day. Research studies at Stanford, Yale, Harvard, and Columbia have also shown gratitude journaling to **improve productivity**, **strengthen relationships**, and **reduce anxiety/depression**. If you'd like to learn more, feel free to head to wethehappyclub.com/research.

This Journal:

This journal features a few activities that we'll briefly motivate below. Feel free to run with the questions as you'd like! :) An entry only takes a max of 5 minutes to fill out.

3 Highlights: This question is intended as a space for you to **note** the highs of the past day as both a primer for the future activities and way for you to keep record of life events.

I am feeling excited about: This question is intended as a space for you to **anchor** your life around things that bring you joy. Reflection around this question provides insight around personal fulfillment.

One thing I love about myself is: This question is intended as a space for **self-love**. You are enough and deserve to be loved - a daily affirmation helps reinforce that!

Weekly Challenges: The weekly challenges are intended to be completed every 5 entries. Feel free to cut them out and keep them some place visible so you follow through on the challenge!

Gratitude Journaling Tips:

Emmons, a professor at the University of California, Davis, shared these research-based tips for reaping the greatest psychological rewards from your gratitude journal.

1. **Go for depth over breadth:** Elaborating in detail about a particular thing for which you're grateful carries more benefits than a superficial list of many things.
2. **Get personal:** Focusing on *people* to whom you are grateful has more of an impact than focusing on *things* for which you are grateful.
3. **Try Subtraction:** One effective way of stimulating gratitude is to reflect on what your life would be like *without* certain blessings, rather than just tallying up all those good things.

Habit Building Tools:

Building a new habit into what may already be a busy schedule can be tough. A few recommendations that I've found particularly helpful....

1. Journal at the **same time** and **place** every day. Many people gratitude journal either first thing when they wake up or right before sleeping.
2. Find a **gratitude accountability partner**. Text/Call someone **right now** you know will keep you accountable. Let said person know you're starting to gratitude journal and ask them check-in.
3. Text "gratitude" to (650) 492 -7201. You will be greeted by Archie the bot who can send you daily reminders, cute gifs, and prompt weekly reflections.
4. **Sticker** the top left square every time you finish an entry! :)
5. If you journal for 21 days, gratitude journaling will be a habit! Identify a reward you will treat yourself with after 21 entries.

My Reward: _____

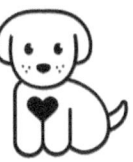

Sticker
Square

Date ____ / ____ / ____

Highlights of the past day?

1. _____
2. _____
3. _____

I am grateful for...

1. _____
   _____

2. _____
   _____

3. _____
   _____

I am feeling excited about...

1. _____
2. _____
3. _____

One thing I love about myself is...

_____

"You must not let anyone define your limits because of where you
come from. Your only limit is your soul." – Ratatouille

Date ___ / ___ / ____

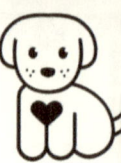

Highlights of the past day?

1. _____
2. _____
3. _____

I am grateful for...

1. _____
   _____

2. _____
   _____

3. _____
   _____

I am feeling excited about...

1. _____
2. _____
3. _____

One thing I love about myself is...

_____

"You yourself, as much as anybody in the entire universe, deserve
your love and affection" – Buddha

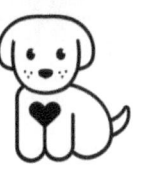

Highlights of the past day?

1. _____
2. _____
3. _____

I am grateful for...

1. _____
_____

2. _____
_____

3. _____
_____

I am feeling excited about...

1. _____
2. _____
3. _____

One thing I love about myself is...

_____

"The best day of your life is the one on which you decide your life is your own. No apologies or excuses. No one to lean on, rely on, or blame. The gift is yours – it is an amazing journey – and you alone are responsible for the quality of it. This is the day your life really begins." – Bob Moawad

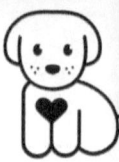

Sticker Square

Date ___ / ___ / ____

Highlights of the past day?

1. _____
2. _____
3. _____

I am grateful for...

1. _____

_____

2. _____

_____

3. _____

_____

I am feeling excited about...

1. _____
2. _____
3. _____

One thing I love about myself is...

_____

"Never be bullied into silence. Never allow yourself to be made a victim. Accept no one's definition of your life, but define yourself." – Harvey Fierstein

Date ___ / ___ / ____

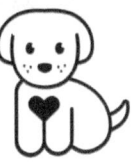

Highlights of the past day?

1. _____
2. _____
3. _____

I am grateful for...

1. _____
   _____

2. _____
   _____

3. _____
   _____

I am feeling excited about...

1. _____
2. _____
3. _____

One thing I love about myself is...

_____

"Until you value yourself, you won't value your time. Until you value
your time, you will not do anything with it." – M. Scott Peck

Weekly Challenge #1

Spread some love and
write a note to someone
who makes you smile. :)

I'm writing to _____

Completion Date: __/__/__

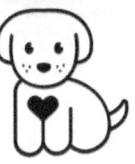

Sticker Square

Date ___ / ___ / ___

Highlights of the past day?

1. _____
2. _____
3. _____

I am grateful for...

1. _____
   _____

2. _____
   _____

3. _____
   _____

I am feeling excited about...

1. _____
2. _____
3. _____

One thing I love about myself is...

_____

"Love yourself first and everything else falls into line. You really have to love yourself to get anything done in this world." – Lucille Ball

Date ___ / ___ / ____

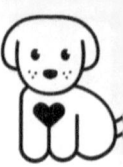

Highlights of the past day?

1. _____
2. _____
3. _____

I am grateful for...

1. _____

_____

2. _____

_____

3. _____

_____

I am feeling excited about...

1. _____
2. _____
3. _____

One thing I love about myself is...

_____

"If only you could sense how important you are to the lives of those you meet; how important you can be to people you may never even dream of. There is something of yourself that you leave at every meeting with another person." – Fred Rogers

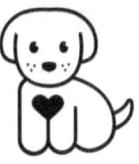

Highlights of the past day?

1. _____
2. _____
3. _____

I am grateful for...

1. _____

   _____

2. _____

   _____

3. _____

   _____

I am feeling excited about...

1. _____
2. _____
3. _____

One thing I love about myself is...

_____

"What lies behind us and what lies before us are tiny matters
compared to what lies within us." – Ralph Waldo Emerson

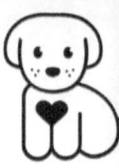

Highlights of the past day?

1. _____
2. _____
3. _____

I am grateful for...

1. _____
_____

2. _____
_____

3. _____
_____

I am feeling excited about...

1. _____
2. _____
3. _____

One thing I love about myself is...

_____

"When you recover or discover something that nourishes your soul and brings joy, care enough about yourself to make room for it in your life." – Jean Shinoda Bolen

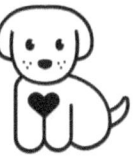

Highlights of the past day?

1. _____
2. _____
3. _____

I am grateful for...

1. _____

_____

2. _____

_____

3. _____

_____

I am feeling excited about...

1. _____
2. _____
3. _____

One thing I love about myself is...

_____

"Why should we worry about what others think of us, do we have more confidence in their opinions than we do our own?" – Brigham Young

Weekly Challenge #2

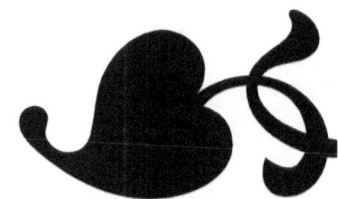

Give the snuggest of hugs to one of your family members.

I gave a hug to _____

Completion Date: __/__/__

Date ___ / ___ / ___

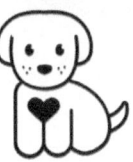

Highlights of the past day?

1. _____
2. _____
3. _____

I am grateful for...

1. _____
   _____

2. _____
   _____

3. _____
   _____

I am feeling excited about...

1. _____
2. _____
3. _____

One thing I love about myself is...

_____

"To love oneself is the beginning of a life-long romance" – Oscar
Wilde

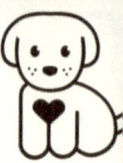

Sticker Square

Date ___ / ___ / ____

Highlights of the past day?

1. _____
2. _____
3. _____

I am grateful for...

1. _____
_____

2. _____
_____

3. _____
_____

I am feeling excited about...

1. _____
2. _____
3. _____

One thing I love about myself is...

_____

"Be faithful to that which exists within yourself." – André Gide

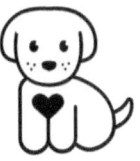

Highlights of the past day?

1. _____
2. _____
3. _____

I am grateful for...

1. _____

   _____

2. _____

   _____

3. _____

   _____

I am feeling excited about...

1. _____
2. _____
3. _____

One thing I love about myself is...

_____

"Who looks outside, dreams; who looks inside, awakes." – Carl

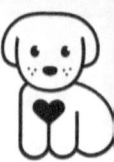

Highlights of the past day?

1. _____
2. _____
3. _____

I am grateful for...

1. _____

_____

2. _____

_____

3. _____

_____

I am feeling excited about...

1. _____
2. _____
3. _____

One thing I love about myself is...

_____

"I think everybody's weird. We should all celebrate our individuality
and not be embarrassed or ashamed of it." – Johnny Depp

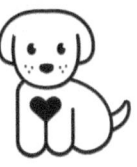

Highlights of the past day?

1. _____
2. _____
3. _____

I am grateful for...

1. _____

_____

2. _____

_____

3. _____

_____

I am feeling excited about...

1. _____
2. _____
3. _____

One thing I love about myself is...

_____

"Never bend your head. Always hold it high. Look the world straight
in the face." – Helen Keller

Weekly Challenge #3

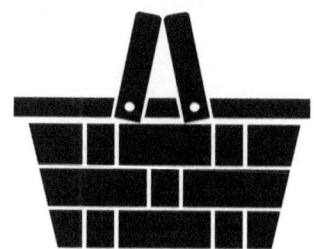

Munch with someone new during a lunch!

I sat with _____

Completion Date: __/__/__

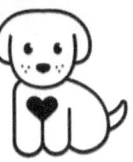

Sticker Square

Date ___ / ___ / _____

Highlights of the past day?

1. _____
2. _____
3. _____

I am grateful for...

1. _____
   _____

2. _____
   _____

3. _____
   _____

I am feeling excited about...

1. _____
2. _____
3. _____

One thing I love about myself is...

_____

"There are days I drop words of comfort on myself like falling leaves and remember that it is enough to be taken care of by myself." – Brian Andreas

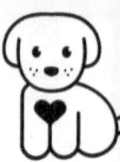

Highlights of the past day?

1. _____
2. _____
3. _____

I am grateful for...

1. _____

_____

2. _____

_____

3. _____

_____

I am feeling excited about...

1. _____
2. _____
3. _____

One thing I love about myself is...

_____

"There is nothing noble about being superior to some other man.
The true nobility is in being superior to your previous self." – Hindu
Proverb

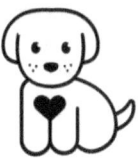

Highlights of the past day?

1. _____
2. _____
3. _____

I am grateful for...

1. _____

_____

2. _____

_____

3. _____

_____

I am feeling excited about...

1. _____
2. _____
3. _____

One thing I love about myself is...

_____

"Act as if what you do makes a difference. It does." – William James

Sticker
Square

Date ___ / ___ / ____

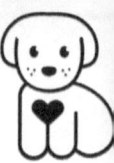

Highlights of the past day?

1. _____
2. _____
3. _____

I am grateful for...

1. _____

   _____

2. _____

   _____

3. _____

   _____

I am feeling excited about...

1. _____
2. _____
3. _____

One thing I love about myself is...

_____

"You are very powerful, provided you know how powerful you are."
– Yogi Bhajan

Date ___ / ___ / ___

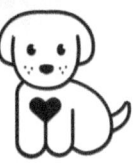

Highlights of the past day?

1. _____
2. _____
3. _____

I am grateful for...

1. _____

   _____

2. _____

   _____

3. _____

   _____

I am feeling excited about...

1. _____
2. _____
3. _____

One thing I love about myself is...

_____

"No matter how your heart is grieving, If you keep on believing, the
dream that you wish will come true." – Cinderella

Weekly Challenge #4

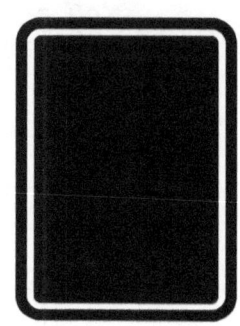

Be a doll and hold the door open for someone at least once!

Completion Date: __/__/__

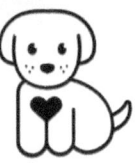

Highlights of the past day?

1. _____
2. _____
3. _____

I am grateful for...

1. _____

_____

2. _____

_____

3. _____

_____

I am feeling excited about...

1. _____
2. _____
3. _____

One thing I love about myself is...

_____

"Don't ask yourself what the world needs, ask yourself what makes
you come alive. And then go and do that. Because what the world
needs is people who have come alive." – Howard Washington
Thurman

CONGRATULATIONS!!!

You've made it 21 days :)

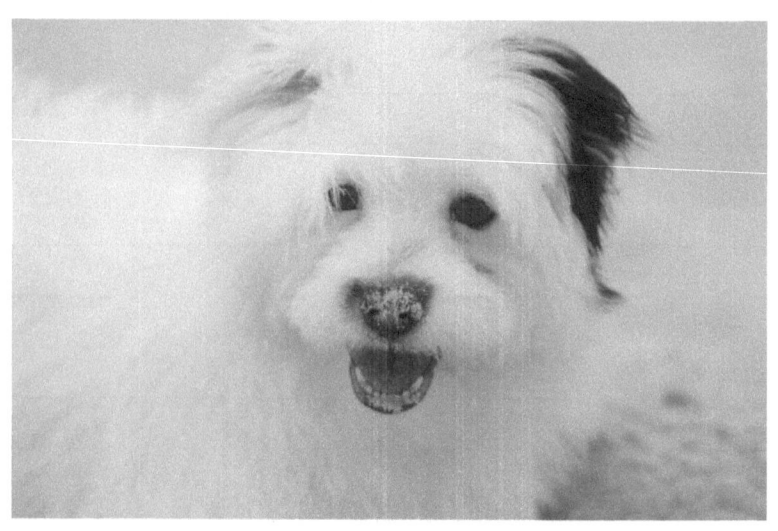

Revisit the reward on Page 5 and treat yourself! :)

Date ___ / ___ / ____

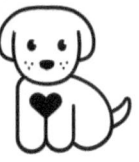

Highlights of the past day?

1. _____

2. _____

3. _____

I am grateful for...

1. _____

_____

2. _____

_____

3. _____

_____

I am feeling excited about...

1. _____

2. _____

3. _____

One thing I love about myself is...

_____

"You're always with yourself, so you might as well enjoy the
company." – Diane Von Furstenberg

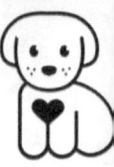

Highlights of the past day?

1. _____
2. _____
3. _____

I am grateful for...

1. _____

_____

2. _____

_____

3. _____

_____

I am feeling excited about...

1. _____
2. _____
3. _____

One thing I love about myself is...

_____

"The best and most beautiful things in the world cannot be seen or even touched - they must be felt with the heart" - Helen Keller

Date ___ / ___ / ___

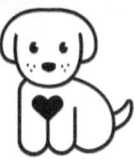

Highlights of the past day?

1. _____
2. _____
3. _____

I am grateful for...

1. _____
   _____

2. _____
   _____

3. _____
   _____

I am feeling excited about...

1. _____
2. _____
3. _____

One thing I love about myself is...

_____

"If we did the things we are capable of, we would astound ourselves" - Thomas Edison

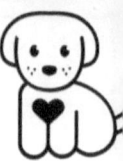

Highlights of the past day?

1. _____
2. _____
3. _____

I am grateful for...

1. _____

_____

2. _____

_____

3. _____

_____

I am feeling excited about...

1. _____
2. _____
3. _____

One thing I love about myself is...

_____

"It is during our darkest moments that we must focus to see the
light" - Aristotle

Weekly Challenge #5

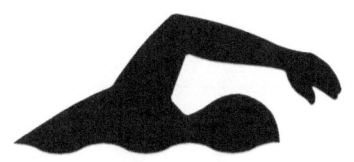

Go outside and do an activity you really love for at least 30 minutes!

Completion Date: __/__/__

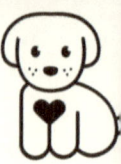

Sticker Square

Date ___ / ___ / ___

Highlights of the past day?

1. _____
2. _____
3. _____

I am grateful for...

1. _____
_____

2. _____
_____

3. _____
_____

I am feeling excited about...

1. _____
2. _____
3. _____

One thing I love about myself is...

_____

"Try to be a rainbow in someone's cloud" - Maya Angelou

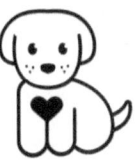

Highlights of the past day?

1. _____
2. _____
3. _____

I am grateful for...

1. _____

_____

2. _____

_____

3. _____

_____

I am feeling excited about...

1. _____
2. _____
3. _____

One thing I love about myself is...

_____

"Don't judge each day by the harvest you reap but by the seeds that you plant." - Robert Louis Stevenson

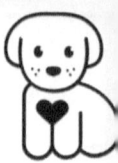

Highlights of the past day?

1. _____
2. _____
3. _____

I am grateful for...

1. _____
_____

2. _____
_____

3. _____
_____

I am feeling excited about...

1. _____
2. _____
3. _____

One thing I love about myself is...

_____

"Nothing is impossible, the word itself says 'I'm possible'!" - Audrey
Hepburn

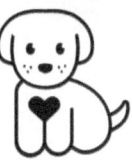

Sticker
Square

Date ___ / ___ / ___

Highlights of the past day?

1. _____
2. _____
3. _____

I am grateful for...

1. _____
   _____

2. _____
   _____

3. _____
   _____

I am feeling excited about...

1. _____
2. _____
3. _____

One thing I love about myself is...

_____

"Where there is love there is life." Mahatma Gandhi

Date ___ / ___ / ____

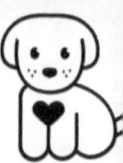

Highlights of the past day?

1. _____
2. _____
3. _____

I am grateful for...

1. _____
_____

2. _____
_____

3. _____
_____

I am feeling excited about...

1. _____
2. _____
3. _____

One thing I love about myself is...

_____

"Feeling gratitude and not expressing it is like wrapping a present
and not giving it." William Arthur Ward

Weekly Challenge #6

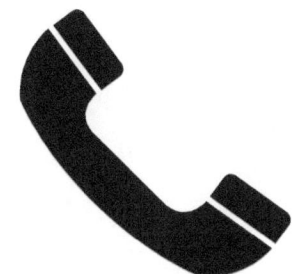

Call a parent/
grandparent and ask
about their favorite
childhood memory!

I called _____

Completion Date: __/__/__

Date ___ / ___ / ____

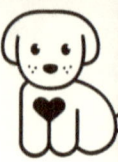

Highlights of the past day?

1. _____
2. _____
3. _____

I am grateful for...

1. _____

_____

2. _____

_____

3. _____

_____

I am feeling excited about...

1. _____
2. _____
3. _____

One thing I love about myself is...

_____

"'Enough' is a feast." Buddhist proverb

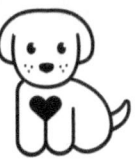

Highlights of the past day?

1. _____
2. _____
3. _____

I am grateful for...

1. _____
_____

2. _____
_____

3. _____
_____

I am feeling excited about...

1. _____
2. _____
3. _____

One thing I love about myself is...

_____

"If you count all your assets, you always show a profit." Robert
Quillen

Date ___ / ___ / ____

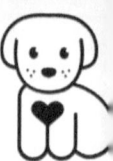

Highlights of the past day?

1. _____
2. _____
3. _____

I am grateful for...

1. _____

_____

2. _____

_____

3. _____

_____

I am feeling excited about...

1. _____
2. _____
3. _____

One thing I love about myself is...

_____

"I would maintain that thanks are the highest form of thought; and that gratitude is happiness doubled by wonder." G.K. Chesterton

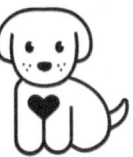

Highlights of the past day?

1. _____
2. _____
3. _____

I am grateful for...

1. _____
   _____

2. _____
   _____

3. _____
   _____

I am feeling excited about...

1. _____
2. _____
3. _____

One thing I love about myself is...

_____

"Enjoy the little things, for one day you may look back and realize
they were the big things." Robert Brault

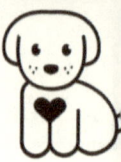

Highlights of the past day?

1. _____
2. _____
3. _____

I am grateful for...

1. _____

_____

2. _____

_____

3. _____

_____

I am feeling excited about...

1. _____
2. _____
3. _____

One thing I love about myself is...

_____

"As we express our gratitude, we must never forget that the highest appreciation is not to utter words but to live by them." John F. Kennedy

Weekly Challenge #7

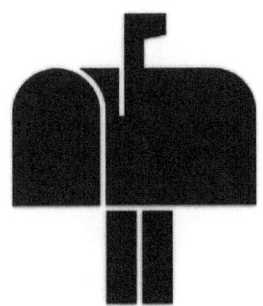

Leave a thank you note
for your mail carrier. :)

Completion Date: __/__/__

Date ___ / ___ / ____

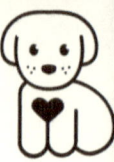

Highlights of the past day?

1. _____
2. _____
3. _____

I am grateful for...

1. _____

_____

2. _____

_____

3. _____

_____

I am feeling excited about...

1. _____
2. _____
3. _____

One thing I love about myself is...

_____

"Acknowledging the good that you already have in your life is the
foundation for all abundance." Eckhart Tolle

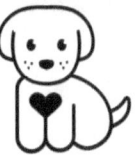

Sticker Square

Date ___ / ___ / ___

Highlights of the past day?

1. _____
2. _____
3. _____

I am grateful for...

1. _____
_____

2. _____
_____

3. _____
_____

I am feeling excited about...

1. _____
2. _____
3. _____

One thing I love about myself is...

_____

"Gratitude turns what we have into enough, and more. It turns
denial into acceptance, chaos into order, confusion into clarity...it
makes sense of our past, brings peace for today, and creates a vision
for tomorrow." Melody Beattie

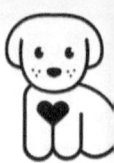

Sticker Square

Date ___ / ___ / ____

Highlights of the past day?

1. _____
2. _____
3. _____

I am grateful for...

1. _____

_____

2. _____

_____

3. _____

_____

I am feeling excited about...

1. _____
2. _____
3. _____

One thing I love about myself is...

_____

"Gratitude is a currency that we can mint for ourselves, and spend
without fear of bankruptcy." Fred De Witt Van Amburgh

Date ___ / ___ / ____

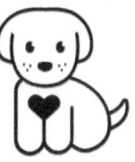

Highlights of the past day?

1. _____
2. _____
3. _____

I am grateful for...

1. _____
   _____

2. _____
   _____

3. _____
   _____

I am feeling excited about...

1. _____
2. _____
3. _____

One thing I love about myself is...

_____

"The way to develop the best that is in a person is by appreciation
and encouragement." Charles Schwab

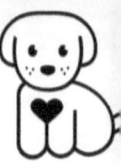

Highlights of the past day?

1. _____
2. _____
3. _____

I am grateful for...

1. _____

_____

2. _____

_____

3. _____

_____

I am feeling excited about...

1. _____
2. _____
3. _____

One thing I love about myself is...

_____

"At times, our own light goes out and is rekindled by a spark from
another person. Each of us has cause to think with deep gratitude of
those who have lighted the flame within us." Albert Schweitzer

Weekly Challenge #8

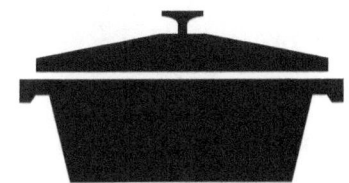

Help make a
scrumptious dinner at
least once this week!

I made dinner with _____
Completion Date: __/__/__

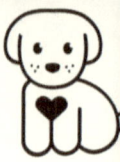

Sticker
Square

Date ___ / ___ / ____

Highlights of the past day?

1. _____
2. _____
3. _____

I am grateful for...

1. _____

_____

2. _____

_____

3. _____

_____

I am feeling excited about...

1. _____
2. _____
3. _____

One thing I love about myself is...

_____

"Be thankful for what you have; you'll end up having more. If you concentrate on what you don't have, you will never, ever have enough." Oprah Winfrey

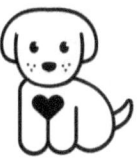

Date ___ / ___ / ___

Highlights of the past day?

1. _____
2. _____
3. _____

I am grateful for...

1. _____

_____

2. _____

_____

3. _____

_____

I am feeling excited about...

1. _____
2. _____
3. _____

One thing I love about myself is...

_____

"You cannot do a kindness too soon because you never know how
soon it will be too late." Ralph Waldo Emerson

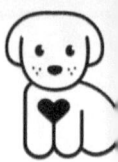

Highlights of the past day?

1. _____
2. _____
3. _____

I am grateful for...

1. _____

_____

2. _____

_____

3. _____

_____

I am feeling excited about...

1. _____
2. _____
3. _____

One thing I love about myself is...

_____

"When I started counting my blessings, my whole life turned
around." Willie Nelson

Date ___ / ___ / ___

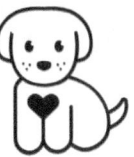

Highlights of the past day?

1. _____
2. _____
3. _____

I am grateful for...

1. _____

_____

2. _____

_____

3. _____

_____

I am feeling excited about...

1. _____
2. _____
3. _____

One thing I love about myself is...

_____

"Things turn out best for people who make the best of the way things turn out." John Wooden

Date ___ / ___ / ____

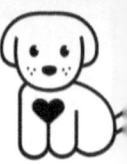

Highlights of the past day?

1. _____
2. _____
3. _____

I am grateful for...

1. _____

_____

2. _____

_____

3. _____

_____

I am feeling excited about...

1. _____
2. _____
3. _____

One thing I love about myself is...

_____

"Piglet noticed that even though he had a very small heart, it could
hold a rather large amount of gratitude." A.A. Milne

Weekly Challenge #9

Show your beautiful smile
to at least 10 people
in passing this week.

Completion Date: __/__/__

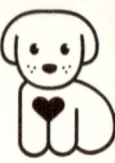

Highlights of the past day?

1. _____
2. _____
3. _____

I am grateful for...

1. _____

_____

2. _____

_____

3. _____

_____

I am feeling excited about...

1. _____
2. _____
3. _____

One thing I love about myself is...

_____

"You yourself, as much as anybody in the entire universe, deserve your love and affection" – Buddha

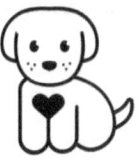

Sticker Square

Date ___ / ___ / ____

Highlights of the past day?

1. _____
2. _____
3. _____

I am grateful for...

1. _____
   _____

2. _____
   _____

3. _____
   _____

I am feeling excited about...

1. _____
2. _____
3. _____

One thing I love about myself is...

_____

"In ordinary life, we hardly realize that we receive a great deal more than we give, and that it is only with gratitude that life becomes rich." Dietrich Bonhoeffer

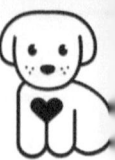

Sticker Square

Date ___ / ___ / ____

Highlights of the past day?

1. _____
2. _____
3. _____

I am grateful for...

1. _____
   _____

2. _____
   _____

3. _____
   _____

I am feeling excited about...

1. _____
2. _____
3. _____

One thing I love about myself is...

_____

"Gratitude also opens your eyes to the limitless potential of the universe, while dissatisfaction closes your eyes to it." Stephen Richards

Sticker
Square

Date ___ / ___ / ___

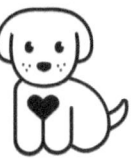

Highlights of the past day?

1. _____
2. _____
3. _____

I am grateful for...

1. _____
   _____

2. _____
   _____

3. _____
   _____

I am feeling excited about...

1. _____
2. _____
3. _____

One thing I love about myself is...

_____

"In life, one has a choice to take one of two paths: to wait for some special day--or to celebrate each special day." Rasheed Ogunlaru

Date ___ / ___ / ___

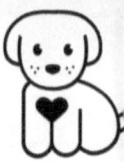

Highlights of the past day?

1. _____
2. _____
3. _____

I am grateful for...

1. _____

   _____

2. _____

   _____

3. _____

   _____

I am feeling excited about...

1. _____
2. _____
3. _____

One thing I love about myself is...

_____

"This a wonderful day. I've never seen this one before." Maya
Angelou

Weekly Challenge #10

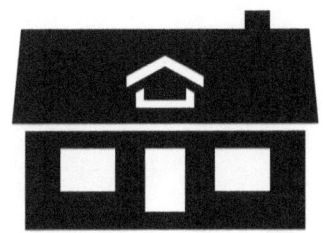

Channel those elf powers
and do someone else's
chores. :)

My chore was _____

Completion Date: __/__/__

Sticker
Square

Date ___ / ___ / ___

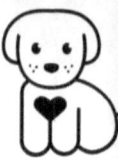

Highlights of the past day?

1. _____
2. _____
3. _____

I am grateful for...

1. _____
_____

2. _____
_____

3. _____
_____

I am feeling excited about...

1. _____
2. _____
3. _____

One thing I love about myself is...

_____

"In today's rush we all think too much - seek too much - want too much - and forget about the joy of just being." ~ Eckhart Tolle

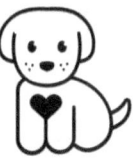

Sticker
Square

Date ___ / ___ / ___

Highlights of the past day?

1. _____
2. _____
3. _____

I am grateful for...

1. _____
   _____

2. _____
   _____

3. _____
   _____

I am feeling excited about...

1. _____
2. _____
3. _____

One thing I love about myself is...

_____

"There is no way to happiness, happiness is the way." ~ Thich Nhat
Hanh

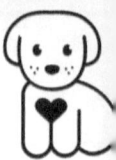

Highlights of the past day?

1. _____
2. _____
3. _____

I am grateful for...

1. _____

_____

2. _____

_____

3. _____

_____

I am feeling excited about...

1. _____
2. _____
3. _____

One thing I love about myself is...

_____

"If we learn to open our hearts, anyone, including the people who
drive us crazy, can be our teacher." ~ Pema Chodron

Date ___ / ___ / ___

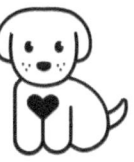

Highlights of the past day?

1. _____
2. _____
3. _____

I am grateful for...

1. _____
   _____

2. _____
   _____

3. _____
   _____

I am feeling excited about...

1. _____
2. _____
3. _____

One thing I love about myself is...

_____

"The pessimist sees difficulty in every opportunity. The optimist sees the opportunity in every difficulty." -Winston Churchill

Date ___ / ___ / ____

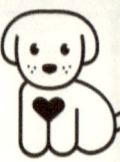

Highlights of the past day?

1. _____
2. _____
3. _____

I am grateful for...

1. _____

_____

2. _____

_____

3. _____

_____

I am feeling excited about...

1. _____
2. _____
3. _____

One thing I love about myself is...

_____

"It's not whether you get knocked down, it's whether you get up." –
Vince Lombardi

Weekly Challenge #11

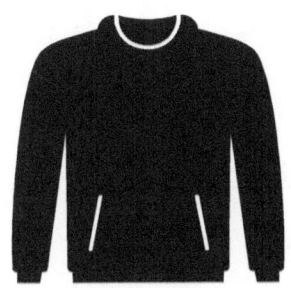

Shake off those overgrown clothes and donate them to a local charity!

I donated to _____

Completion Date: __/__/__

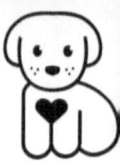

Highlights of the past day?

1. _____
2. _____
3. _____

I am grateful for...

1. _____

_____

2. _____

_____

3. _____

_____

I am feeling excited about...

1. _____
2. _____
3. _____

One thing I love about myself is...

_____

"People who are crazy enough to think they can change the world,
are the ones that do"- Rob Siltanen

Date ___ / ___ / ___

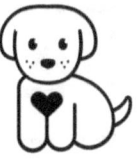

Highlights of the past day?

1. _____
2. _____
3. _____

I am grateful for...

1. _____
_____

2. _____
_____

3. _____
_____

I am feeling excited about...

1. _____
2. _____
3. _____

One thing I love about myself is...

_____

"We may encounter many defeats but we must not be defeated."
- Maya Angelou

Date ___ / ___ / ____

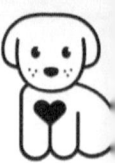

Highlights of the past day?

1. _____
2. _____
3. _____

I am grateful for...

1. _____

_____

2. _____

_____

3. _____

_____

I am feeling excited about...

1. _____
2. _____
3. _____

One thing I love about myself is...

_____

"Where you think you can or think you can't, you're right."- Henry
Ford

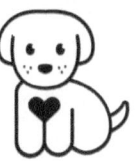

Highlights of the past day?

1. _____
2. _____
3. _____

I am grateful for...

1. _____

_____

2. _____

_____

3. _____

_____

I am feeling excited about...

1. _____
2. _____
3. _____

One thing I love about myself is...

_____

"Do what you can with all you have, wherever you are."- Theodore
Roosevelt

Date ___ / ___ / ____

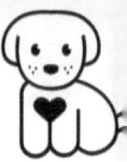

Highlights of the past day?

1. _____
2. _____
3. _____

I am grateful for...

1. _____

   _____

2. _____

   _____

3. _____

   _____

I am feeling excited about...

1. _____
2. _____
3. _____

One thing I love about myself is...

_____

"Discouragement and failure are two of the surest stepping stones
to success." ~Dale Carnegie

Weekly Challenge #12

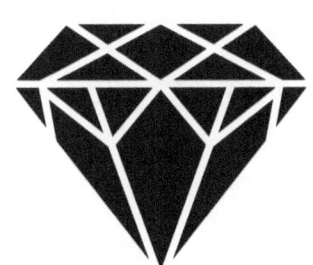

Make someone's day by letting them know how special they are to you!

I let _____ know

Completion Date: __/__/__

Date ___ / ___ / ____

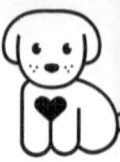

Highlights of the past day?

1. _____
2. _____
3. _____

I am grateful for...

1. _____

_____

2. _____

_____

3. _____

_____

I am feeling excited about...

1. _____
2. _____
3. _____

One thing I love about myself is...

_____

"Once you choose hope, anything's possible." ~Christopher Reeve

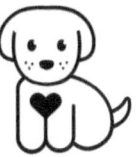

Sticker
Square

Date ___ / ___ / ____

Highlights of the past day?

1. _____
2. _____
3. _____

I am grateful for...

1. _____

_____

2. _____

_____

3. _____

_____

I am feeling excited about...

1. _____
2. _____
3. _____

One thing I love about myself is...

_____

"Most great people have attained their greatest success one step
beyond their greatest failure." ~Napoleon Hill

Date ___ / ___ / ____

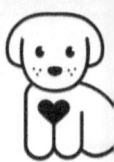

Highlights of the past day?

1. _____
2. _____
3. _____

I am grateful for...

1. _____

_____

2. _____

_____

3. _____

_____

I am feeling excited about...

1. _____
2. _____
3. _____

One thing I love about myself is...

_____

"The best way to predict the future is to create it." ~Abraham Lincoln

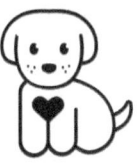

Sticker Square

Date ___ / ___ / ____

Highlights of the past day?

1. _____
2. _____
3. _____

I am grateful for...

1. _____

_____

2. _____

_____

3. _____

_____

I am feeling excited about...

1. _____
2. _____
3. _____

One thing I love about myself is...

_____

"The first step is you have to say that you can" ~Will Smith

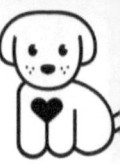

Sticker Square

Date ___ / ___ / ___

Highlights of the past day?

1. _____
2. _____
3. _____

I am grateful for...

1. _____

_____

2. _____

_____

3. _____

_____

I am feeling excited about...

1. _____
2. _____
3. _____

One thing I love about myself is...

_____

"Only those who dare to fail greatly can ever achieve greatly."
~Robert F. Kennedy

Weekly Challenge #13

Read a book you've always wanted to but never got the time to!

I read: _____

Completion Date: __/__/__

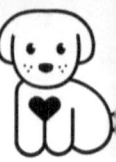

Highlights of the past day?

1. _____
2. _____
3. _____

I am grateful for...

1. _____

   _____

2. _____

   _____

3. _____

   _____

I am feeling excited about...

1. _____
2. _____
3. _____

One thing I love about myself is...

_____

"If I persist long enough I will win." ~Og Mandino

Date ___ / ___ / ___

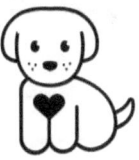

Highlights of the past day?

1. _____
2. _____
3. _____

I am grateful for...

1. _____

_____

2. _____

_____

3. _____

_____

I am feeling excited about...

1. _____
2. _____
3. _____

One thing I love about myself is...

_____

"The dreamers are the saviors of the world." ~James Allen

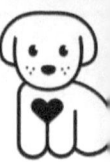

Highlights of the past day?

1. _____
2. _____
3. _____

I am grateful for...

1. _____
   _____

2. _____
   _____

3. _____
   _____

I am feeling excited about...

1. _____
2. _____
3. _____

One thing I love about myself is...

_____

"I've failed over and over and over again in my life. And that is why I succeed." ~Michael Jordan

Date ___ / ___ / ____

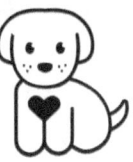

Highlights of the past day?

1. _____
2. _____
3. _____

I am grateful for...

1. _____
_____

2. _____
_____

3. _____
_____

I am feeling excited about...

1. _____
2. _____
3. _____

One thing I love about myself is...

_____

"If there is no struggle, there is no progress." ~Frederick Douglass

Date ___ / ___ / ____

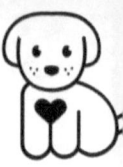

Highlights of the past day?

1. _____
2. _____
3. _____

I am grateful for...

1. _____

_____

2. _____

_____

3. _____

_____

I am feeling excited about...

1. _____
2. _____
3. _____

One thing I love about myself is...

_____

"Rise above the storm and you will find the sunshine." ~Mario Fernandez

Weekly Challenge #14

Tell a family member how much you love them.

I told _____

Completion Date: __/__/__

Date ____ / ____ / ____

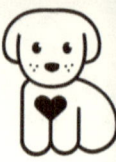

Highlights of the past day?

1. _____
2. _____
3. _____

I am grateful for...

1. _____

_____

2. _____

_____

3. _____

_____

I am feeling excited about...

1. _____
2. _____
3. _____

One thing I love about myself is...

_____

"The best is yet to be." ~Robert Browning

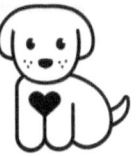

Sticker
Square

Date ___ / ___ / ____

Highlights of the past day?

1. _____
2. _____
3. _____

I am grateful for...

1. _____
_____

2. _____
_____

3. _____
_____

I am feeling excited about...

1. _____
2. _____
3. _____

One thing I love about myself is...

_____

"Life has no limitations, except the ones you make." ~Les Brown

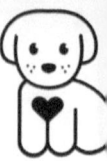

Highlights of the past day?

1. _____

2. _____

3. _____

I am grateful for...

1. _____

   _____

2. _____

   _____

3. _____

   _____

I am feeling excited about...

1. _____

2. _____

3. _____

One thing I love about myself is...

_____

"The world is more malleable than you think and it's waiting for you
to hammer it into shape." ~Bono

Date ___ / ___ / ___

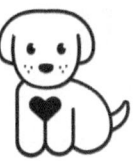

Highlights of the past day?

1. _____
2. _____
3. _____

I am grateful for...

1. _____
   _____

2. _____
   _____

3. _____
   _____

I am feeling excited about...

1. _____
2. _____
3. _____

One thing I love about myself is...

_____

"It always seems impossible until it's done." ~Nelson Mandela

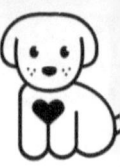

Sticker Square

Date ___ / ___ / ____

Highlights of the past day?

1. _____
2. _____
3. _____

I am grateful for...

1. _____
_____

2. _____
_____

3. _____
_____

I am feeling excited about...

1. _____
2. _____
3. _____

One thing I love about myself is...

_____

"All life is an experiment. The more experiments you make, the better." ~Ralph Waldo Emerson

Weekly Challenge #15

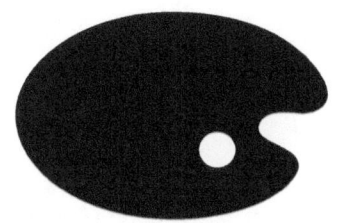

Paint/draw/color your
happiest place.

I painted _____

Completion Date: __/__/__

Date ___ / ___ / ____

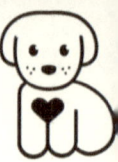

Highlights of the past day?

1. _____
2. _____
3. _____

I am grateful for...

1. _____
   _____

2. _____
   _____

3. _____
   _____

I am feeling excited about...

1. _____
2. _____
3. _____

One thing I love about myself is...

_____

"Yesterday is history, tomorrow is a mystery, but today is a gift...
that's why we call it the present" ~ Kung Fu Panda

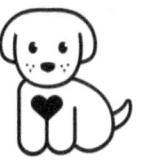

Highlights of the past day?

1. _____
2. _____
3. _____

I am grateful for...

1. _____
_____

2. _____
_____

3. _____
_____

I am feeling excited about...

1. _____
2. _____
3. _____

One thing I love about myself is...

_____

"Life is the dancer and you're the dance" - Eckhart Tolle

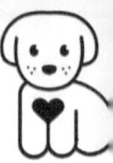

Highlights of the past day?

1. _____
2. _____
3. _____

I am grateful for...

1. _____

_____

2. _____

_____

3. _____

_____

I am feeling excited about...

1. _____
2. _____
3. _____

One thing I love about myself is...

_____

"Only in the darkness can you see the stars" ~ Martin Luther King Jr.

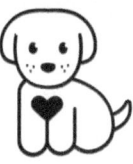

Sticker
Square

Date ___ / ___ / ____

Highlights of the past day?

1. _____
2. _____
3. _____

I am grateful for...

1. _____
   _____

2. _____
   _____

3. _____
   _____

I am feeling excited about...

1. _____
2. _____
3. _____

One thing I love about myself is...

_____

"You can't stop waves but you can learn to swim" ~ Jon Kabat Zim

Date ___ / ___ / ___

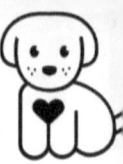

Highlights of the past day?

1. _____
2. _____
3. _____

I am grateful for...

1. _____

_____

2. _____

_____

3. _____

_____

I am feeling excited about...

1. _____
2. _____
3. _____

One thing I love about myself is...

_____

"Just when the caterpillar thought its world was over, it became a butterfly"

Weekly Challenge #16

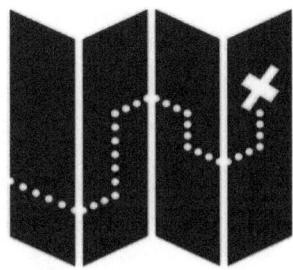

Take time to reflect on what you've written in your journal so far.

Completion Date: __/__/__

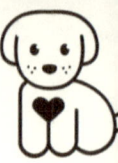

Sticker
Square

Date ___ / ___ / ____

Highlights of the past day?

1. _____
2. _____
3. _____

I am grateful for...

1. _____

_____

2. _____

_____

3. _____

_____

I am feeling excited about...

1. _____
2. _____
3. _____

One thing I love about myself is...

_____

"Don't underestimate the value of doing nothing, of just going
along, listening to all the things you can't hear, and not bothering."
Winnie the Pooh

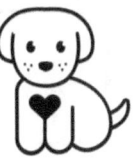

Sticker Square

Date ___ / ___ / ___

Highlights of the past day?

1. _____
2. _____
3. _____

I am grateful for...

1. _____
_____

2. _____
_____

3. _____
_____

I am feeling excited about...

1. _____
2. _____
3. _____

One thing I love about myself is...

_____

"That's the real trouble with the world, too many people grow up" ~
Walt Disney

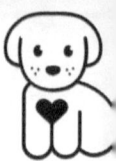

Sticker Square

Date ___ / ___ / ____

Highlights of the past day?

1. _____
2. _____
3. _____

I am grateful for...

1. _____
   _____

2. _____
   _____

3. _____
   _____

I am feeling excited about...

1. _____
2. _____
3. _____

One thing I love about myself is...

_____

"Love is putting someone else's needs before yours." – Frozen

Sticker Square

Date ___ / ___ / _____

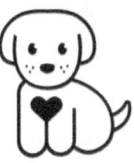

Highlights of the past day?

1. _____
2. _____
3. _____

I am grateful for...

1. _____
_____

2. _____
_____

3. _____
_____

I am feeling excited about...

1. _____
2. _____
3. _____

One thing I love about myself is...

_____

"The flower that blooms in adversity is the most rare and beautiful
of them all." – Mulan

Date ___ / ___ / ____

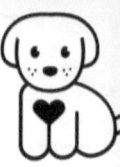

Highlights of the past day?

1. _____

2. _____

3. _____

I am grateful for...

1. _____

_____

2. _____

_____

3. _____

_____

I am feeling excited about...

1. _____

2. _____

3. _____

One thing I love about myself is...

_____

"I was hiding under your porch because I love you." – Up

Weekly Challenge #17

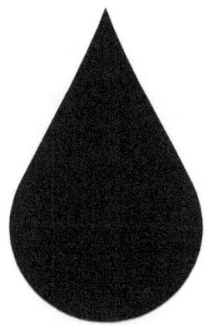

Take <5 minute showers this week to conserve water.

Completion Date: __/__/__

Date ___ / ___ / ____

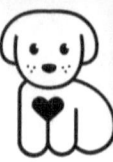

Highlights of the past day?

1. _____
2. _____
3. _____

I am grateful for...

1. _____

_____

2. _____

_____

3. _____

_____

I am feeling excited about...

1. _____
2. _____
3. _____

One thing I love about myself is...

_____

"'Ohana means family, and family means no one gets left behind or
forgotten." – Lilo & Stitch

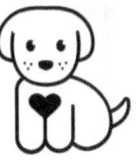

Sticker Square

Date ___ / ___ / ____

Highlights of the past day?

1. _____
2. _____
3. _____

I am grateful for...

1. _____

_____

2. _____

_____

3. _____

_____

I am feeling excited about...

1. _____
2. _____
3. _____

One thing I love about myself is...

_____

"The past can hurt. But the way I see it, you can either run from it, or learn from it." – The Lion King

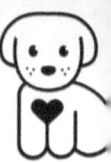

Highlights of the past day?

1. _____
2. _____
3. _____

I am grateful for...

1. _____

_____

2. _____

_____

3. _____

_____

I am feeling excited about...

1. _____
2. _____
3. _____

One thing I love about myself is...

_____

"You're braver than you believe, and stronger than you seem, and smarter than you think." – Winnie the Pooh

Sticker
Square

Date ___ / ___ / ___

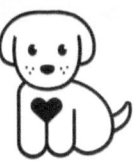

Highlights of the past day?

1. _____
2. _____
3. _____

I am grateful for...

1. _____

_____

2. _____

_____

3. _____

_____

I am feeling excited about...

1. _____
2. _____
3. _____

One thing I love about myself is...

_____

"Our fate lives within us. You only have to be brave enough to see it." – Brave

Date ___ / ___ / ___

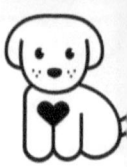

Highlights of the past day?

1. _____
2. _____
3. _____

I am grateful for...

1. _____

   _____

2. _____

   _____

3. _____

   _____

I am feeling excited about...

1. _____
2. _____
3. _____

One thing I love about myself is...

_____

"She warned him not to be deceived by appearances, for beauty is found within." – Beauty and the Beast

Weekly Challenge #18

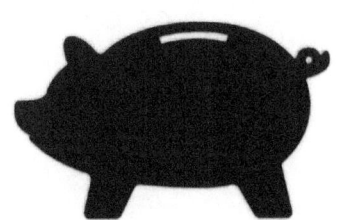

Put on your giving cap and donate to a local charity!

I donated to _____

Completion Date: __/__/__

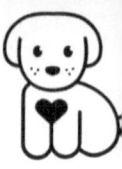

Highlights of the past day?

1. _____
2. _____
3. _____

I am grateful for...

1. _____

_____

2. _____

_____

3. _____

_____

I am feeling excited about...

1. _____
2. _____
3. _____

One thing I love about myself is...

_____

"The very things that hold you down are going to lift you up." –
Timothy Mouse, Dumbo

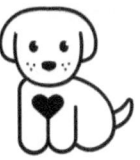

Sticker Square

Date ___ / ___ / ____

Highlights of the past day?

1. _____
2. _____
3. _____

I am grateful for...

1. _____
_____

2. _____
_____

3. _____
_____

I am feeling excited about...

1. _____
2. _____
3. _____

One thing I love about myself is...

_____

"When life gets you down do you wanna know what you've gotta do? Just keep swimming!" – Dory, Finding Nemo

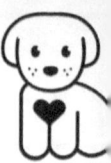

Sticker Square

Date ___ / ___ / ____

Highlights of the past day?

1. _____
2. _____
3. _____

I am grateful for...

1. _____
_____

2. _____
_____

3. _____
_____

I am feeling excited about...

1. _____
2. _____
3. _____

One thing I love about myself is...

_____

"Fairy tales can come true. You gotta make them happen, it all
depends on you." – Tiana, Princess and the Frog

Date ___ / ___ / ____

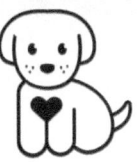

Highlights of the past day?

1. _____
2. _____
3. _____

I am grateful for...

1. _____

_____

2. _____

_____

3. _____

_____

I am feeling excited about...

1. _____
2. _____
3. _____

One thing I love about myself is...

_____

"Do what you feel in your heart to be right — for you'll be criticized anyway. You'll be 'damned if you do, and damned if you don't.'" ~ Eleanor Roosevelt

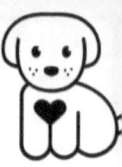

Highlights of the past day?

1. _____
2. _____
3. _____

I am grateful for...

1. _____

_____

2. _____

_____

3. _____

_____

I am feeling excited about...

1. _____
2. _____
3. _____

One thing I love about myself is...

_____

"In matters of style, swim with the current; in matters of principle,
stand like a rock." ~ Thomas Jefferson

Weekly Challenge #19

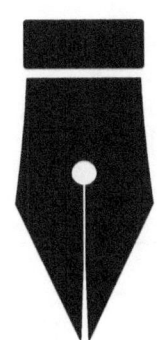

Write and deliver a card for your favorite teacher!

My fave teacher is _____

Completion Date: __/__/__

Date ___ / ___ / ____

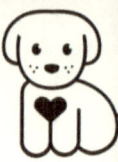

Highlights of the past day?

1. _____
2. _____
3. _____

I am grateful for...

1. _____
   _____

2. _____
   _____

3. _____
   _____

I am feeling excited about...

1. _____
2. _____
3. _____

One thing I love about myself is...

_____

"I've learned from experience that the greater part of our happiness
or misery depends on our dispositions and not on our
circumstances." ~ Martha Washington

Date ___ / ___ / ____

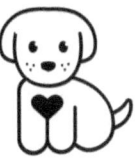

Highlights of the past day?

1. _____
2. _____
3. _____

I am grateful for...

1. _____

   _____

2. _____

   _____

3. _____

   _____

I am feeling excited about...

1. _____
2. _____
3. _____

One thing I love about myself is...

_____

"Challenge yourself with something you know you could never do,
and what you'll find is that you can overcome anything." ~ Anon

Date ___ / ___ / ____

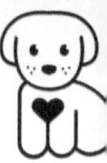

Highlights of the past day?

1. _____
2. _____
3. _____

I am grateful for...

1. _____
_____

2. _____
_____

3. _____
_____

I am feeling excited about...

1. _____
2. _____
3. _____

One thing I love about myself is...

_____

"You cannot shake hands with a clenched fist." ~ Indira Gandhi

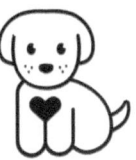

Sticker
Square

Date ___ / ___ / ____

Highlights of the past day?

1. _____
2. _____
3. _____

I am grateful for...

1. _____
   _____

2. _____
   _____

3. _____
   _____

I am feeling excited about...

1. _____
2. _____
3. _____

One thing I love about myself is...

_____

"Darkness cannot drive out darkness: only light can do that. Hate
cannot drive out hate: only love can do that." ~ Martin Luther King
Jr

Date ___ / ___ / ____

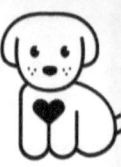

Highlights of the past day?

1. _____
2. _____
3. _____

I am grateful for...

1. _____

_____

2. _____

_____

3. _____

_____

I am feeling excited about...

1. _____
2. _____
3. _____

One thing I love about myself is...

_____

"You yourself, as much as anybody in the entire universe, deserve
your love and affection" – Buddha

Weekly Challenge #20

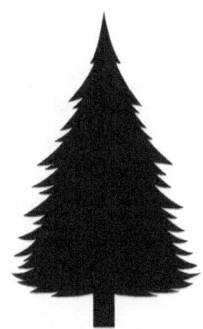

The wilderness must be explored! Go for a hike with an adventurous family member!

I hiked _____

Completion Date: __/__/__

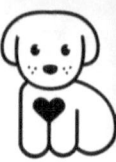

Highlights of the past day?

1. _____
2. _____
3. _____

I am grateful for...

1. _____

_____

2. _____

_____

3. _____

_____

I am feeling excited about...

1. _____
2. _____
3. _____

One thing I love about myself is...

_____

"Aerodynamically, the bumblebee shouldn't be able to fly, but the bumblebee doesn't know that so it goes on flying anyway." ~ Mary Kay Ash

Date ___ / ___ / ____

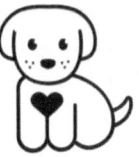

Highlights of the past day?

1. _____
2. _____
3. _____

I am grateful for...

1. _____

_____

2. _____

_____

3. _____

_____

I am feeling excited about...

1. _____
2. _____
3. _____

One thing I love about myself is...

_____

"The real opportunity for success lies within the person and not in
the job." ~ Zig Ziglar

Date ___ / ___ / ____

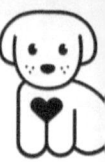

Highlights of the past day?

1. _____
2. _____
3. _____

I am grateful for...

1. _____

_____

2. _____

_____

3. _____

_____

I am feeling excited about...

1. _____
2. _____
3. _____

One thing I love about myself is...

_____

"Love is the emblem of eternity; it confounds all notion of time;
effaces all memory of a beginning, all fear of an end." ~ Germaine
De Stael

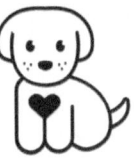

Sticker Square

Date ___ / ___ / ____

Highlights of the past day?

1. _____
2. _____
3. _____

I am grateful for...

1. _____
   _____

2. _____
   _____

3. _____
   _____

I am feeling excited about...

1. _____
2. _____
3. _____

One thing I love about myself is...

_____

"It takes a great deal of courage to stand up to your enemies, but even more to stand up to your friends." ~ JK Rowling

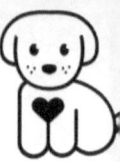

Highlights of the past day?

1. _____
2. _____
3. _____

I am grateful for...

1. _____

_____

2. _____

_____

3. _____

_____

I am feeling excited about...

1. _____
2. _____
3. _____

One thing I love about myself is...

_____

"Nothing else in the world . . . not all the armies . . . is so powerful
as an idea whose time has come." ~ Victor Hugo

Weekly Challenge #21

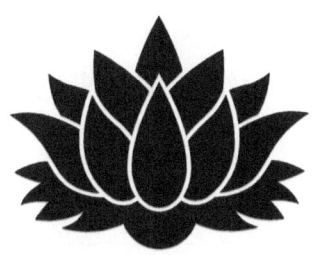

Channel your spiritual energy and practice mindfulness for 5 minutes each morning.

Completion Date: __/__/__

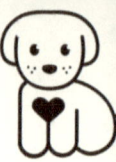

Sticker
Square

Date ___ / ___ / ____

Highlights of the past day?

1. _____
2. _____
3. _____

I am grateful for...

1. _____
   _____

2. _____
   _____

3. _____
   _____

I am feeling excited about...

1. _____
2. _____
3. _____

One thing I love about myself is...

_____

"Friendship is like peeing on yourself: everyone can see it, but only
you get the warm feeling that it brings." ~ Robert Bloch

Sticker
Square

Date ___ / ___ / ____

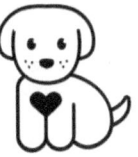

Highlights of the past day?

1. _____
2. _____
3. _____

I am grateful for...

1. _____
   _____

2. _____
   _____

3. _____
   _____

I am feeling excited about...

1. _____
2. _____
3. _____

One thing I love about myself is...

_____

"What is harder than rock, or softer than water? Yet soft water
hollows out hard rock. Persevere." ~ Ovid

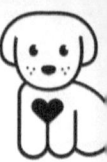

Sticker Square

Date ___ / ___ / ____

Highlights of the past day?

1. _____
2. _____
3. _____

I am grateful for...

1. _____
   _____

2. _____
   _____

3. _____
   _____

I am feeling excited about...

1. _____
2. _____
3. _____

One thing I love about myself is...

_____

"Keep away from people who try to belittle your ambitions. Small people always do that, but the really great make you feel that you, too, can become great." ~ Mark Twain

Date ___ / ___ / ____

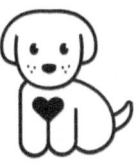

Highlights of the past day?

1. _____
2. _____
3. _____

I am grateful for...

1. _____
   _____

2. _____
   _____

3. _____
   _____

I am feeling excited about...

1. _____
2. _____
3. _____

One thing I love about myself is...

_____

"Stay hungry. Stay foolish." ~ Steward Brand

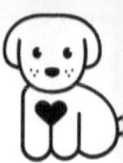

Highlights of the past day?

1. _____
2. _____
3. _____

I am grateful for...

1. _____

_____

2. _____

_____

3. _____

_____

I am feeling excited about...

1. _____
2. _____
3. _____

One thing I love about myself is...

_____

"Don't find fault. Find remedy. Anyone can complain." ~ Henry Ford

Weekly Challenge #22

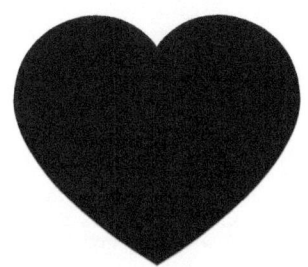

Treat yourself in at least one way this week to practice self-care.

I _____

Completion Date: __/__/__

Date ___ / ___ / ___

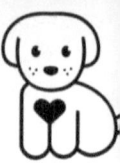

Highlights of the past day?

1. _____
2. _____
3. _____

I am grateful for...

1. _____

   _____

2. _____

   _____

3. _____

   _____

I am feeling excited about...

1. _____
2. _____
3. _____

One thing I love about myself is...

_____

"The future belongs to those who believe in the beauty of their
dreams." ~ Eleanor Roosevelt

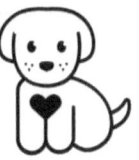

Highlights of the past day?

1. _____
2. _____
3. _____

I am grateful for...

1. _____

_____

2. _____

_____

3. _____

_____

I am feeling excited about...

1. _____
2. _____
3. _____

One thing I love about myself is...

_____

"A mind is like a parachute. It doesn't work if it isn't open." ~ Frank
Zappa

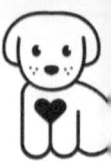

Highlights of the past day?

1. _____
2. _____
3. _____

I am grateful for...

1. _____

_____

2. _____

_____

3. _____

_____

I am feeling excited about...

1. _____
2. _____
3. _____

One thing I love about myself is...

_____

"Failure is simply the opportunity to begin again, this time more
intelligently." ~ Henry Ford

Sticker
Square

Date ___ / ___ / ___

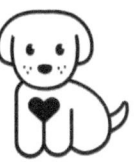

Highlights of the past day?

1. _____
2. _____
3. _____

I am grateful for...

1. _____

_____

2. _____

_____

3. _____

_____

I am feeling excited about...

1. _____
2. _____
3. _____

One thing I love about myself is...

_____

"People will forget what you said. People will forget what you did.
But people will never forget how you made them feel." ~ Maya
Angelou

Date ___ / ___ / ____

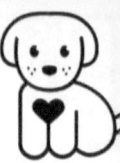

Highlights of the past day?

1. _____
2. _____
3. _____

I am grateful for...

1. _____

_____

2. _____

_____

3. _____

_____

I am feeling excited about...

1. _____
2. _____
3. _____

One thing I love about myself is...

_____

"The man who removes a mountain begins by carrying away small
stones." ~ Chinese Proverb

Weekly Challenge #23

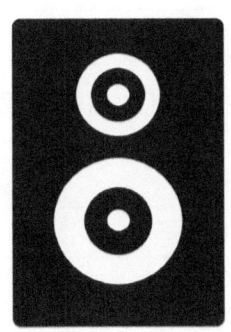

Bust out those moves and have a dance party at home with friends/family!

Completion Date: __/__/__

Date ___ / ___ / ____

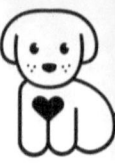

Highlights of the past day?

1. _____
2. _____
3. _____

I am grateful for...

1. _____

_____

2. _____

_____

3. _____

_____

I am feeling excited about...

1. _____
2. _____
3. _____

One thing I love about myself is...

_____

"In between goals is a thing called life, that has to be lived and
enjoyed." ~ Sid Caesar

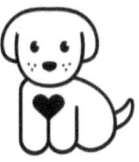

Sticker Square

Date ___ / ___ / ____

Highlights of the past day?

1. _____
2. _____
3. _____

I am grateful for...

1. _____
   _____

2. _____
   _____

3. _____
   _____

I am feeling excited about...

1. _____
2. _____
3. _____

One thing I love about myself is...

_____

"If you want to make your dreams come true, the first thing you
have to do is wake up." ~ J.M Power

Sticker Square

Date ___ / ___ / ___

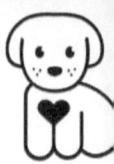

Highlights of the past day?

1. _____
2. _____
3. _____

I am grateful for...

1. _____

_____

2. _____

_____

3. _____

_____

I am feeling excited about...

1. _____
2. _____
3. _____

One thing I love about myself is...

_____

"A ship in harbor is safe, but that is not what ships are built for." ~
John Shed

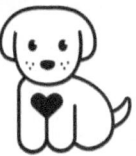

Highlights of the past day?

1. _____
2. _____
3. _____

I am grateful for...

1. _____
_____

2. _____
_____

3. _____
_____

I am feeling excited about...

1. _____
2. _____
3. _____

One thing I love about myself is...

_____

"We could learn a lot from crayons; some are sharp, some are pretty, some are dull, while others bright, some have weird names, but they all have learned to live together in the same box." ~ Robert

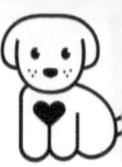

Highlights of the past day?

1. _____
2. _____
3. _____

I am grateful for...

1. _____
_____

2. _____
_____

3. _____
_____

I am feeling excited about...

1. _____
2. _____
3. _____

One thing I love about myself is...

_____

"It is a good thing to be rich and a good thing to be strong, but it is a better thing to be loved by many friends." ~ Euripedes

Weekly Challenge #24

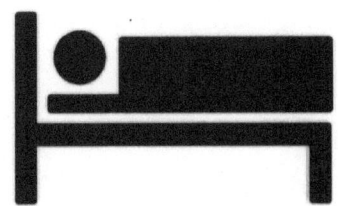

Take special care to catch some zzzzs this week and sleep for at least 7-8 hours!

Completion Date: __/__/__

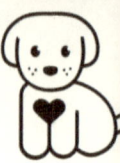

Sticker Square

Date ___ / ___ / ___

Highlights of the past day?

1. _____
2. _____
3. _____

I am grateful for...

1. _____

_____

2. _____

_____

3. _____

_____

I am feeling excited about...

1. _____
2. _____
3. _____

One thing I love about myself is...

_____

"Some cause happiness wherever they go; others, whenever they
go." ~ Oscar Wilde

Sticker
Square

Date ___ / ___ / ___

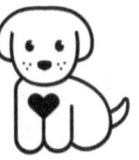

Highlights of the past day?

1. _____
2. _____
3. _____

I am grateful for...

1. _____
_____

2. _____
_____

3. _____
_____

I am feeling excited about...

1. _____
2. _____
3. _____

One thing I love about myself is...

_____

"I'd rather die on my feet, than live upon my knees." ~ Emiliano
Zapata

Date ___ / ___ / ___

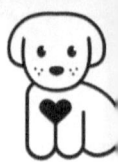

Highlights of the past day?

1. _____
2. _____
3. _____

I am grateful for...

1. _____
_____

2. _____
_____

3. _____
_____

I am feeling excited about...

1. _____
2. _____
3. _____

One thing I love about myself is...

_____

"I am a great believer in luck. The harder I work, the more of it I
seem to have." ~ Coleman Cox

Date ___ / ___ / ___

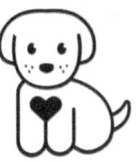

Highlights of the past day?

1. _____
2. _____
3. _____

I am grateful for...

1. _____
_____

2. _____
_____

3. _____
_____

I am feeling excited about...

1. _____
2. _____
3. _____

One thing I love about myself is...

_____

"Love is, above all else, the gift of oneself." ~ Jean Anouilh

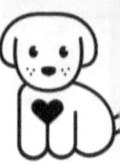

Sticker Square

Date ___ / ___ / ___

Highlights of the past day?

1. _____
2. _____
3. _____

I am grateful for...

1. _____

_____

2. _____

_____

3. _____

_____

I am feeling excited about...

1. _____
2. _____
3. _____

One thing I love about myself is...

_____

"Music expresses that which cannot be said and on which it is impossible to be silent." ~ Victor Hugo

Weekly Challenge #25

Don't watch any TV or movies this week - notice how you feel.

Completion Date: __/__/__

Date ___ / ___ / ____

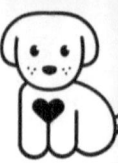

Highlights of the past day?

1. _____
2. _____
3. _____

I am grateful for...

1. _____

_____

2. _____

_____

3. _____

_____

I am feeling excited about...

1. _____
2. _____
3. _____

One thing I love about myself is...

_____

"Being the richest man in the cemetery doesn't matter to me. Going to bed at night saying we've done something wonderful, that's what matters to me." ~ Steve Jobs

Date ___ / ___ / ___

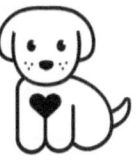

Highlights of the past day?

1. _____

2. _____

3. _____

I am grateful for...

1. _____

_____

2. _____

_____

3. _____

_____

I am feeling excited about...

1. _____

2. _____

3. _____

One thing I love about myself is...

_____

"The best and most beautiful things in the world cannot be seen nor
even touched, but just felt in the heart." ~ Anne Sullivan

Date ___ / ___ / _____

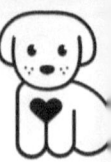

Highlights of the past day?

1. _____
2. _____
3. _____

I am grateful for...

1. _____

_____

2. _____

_____

3. _____

_____

I am feeling excited about...

1. _____
2. _____
3. _____

One thing I love about myself is...

_____

'You can't go back and make a new start, but you can start right now
and make a brand new ending." ~ James Sherman

Date ___ / ___ / ____

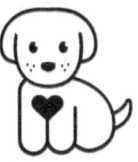

Highlights of the past day?

1. _____
2. _____
3. _____

I am grateful for...

1. _____
   _____

2. _____
   _____

3. _____
   _____

I am feeling excited about...

1. _____
2. _____
3. _____

One thing I love about myself is...

_____

"Life consists not in holding good cards but in playing those you
hold well." ~ Josh Billings

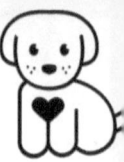

Highlights of the past day?

1. _____
2. _____
3. _____

I am grateful for...

1. _____

_____

2. _____

_____

3. _____

_____

I am feeling excited about...

1. _____
2. _____
3. _____

One thing I love about myself is...

_____

"When you judge another, you do not define them, you define
yourself." ~ Wayne Dyer

Weekly Challenge #26

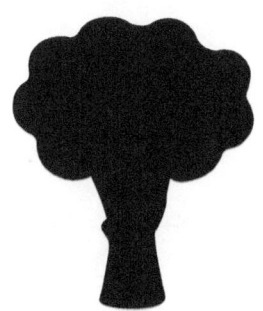

Eat at least one serving of veggies with every meal this week!

Completion Date: __/__/__

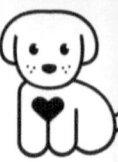

Highlights of the past day?

1. _____
2. _____
3. _____

I am grateful for...

1. _____

_____

2. _____

_____

3. _____

_____

I am feeling excited about...

1. _____
2. _____
3. _____

One thing I love about myself is...

_____

"In the arithmetic of love, one plus one equals everything, and two minus one equals nothing." ~ Mignon Mclaughlin

Date ___ / ___ / ___

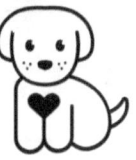

Highlights of the past day?

1. _____
2. _____
3. _____

I am grateful for...

1. _____
_____

2. _____
_____

3. _____
_____

I am feeling excited about...

1. _____
2. _____
3. _____

One thing I love about myself is...

_____

"The cave you fear to enter holds the treasure you seek." ~ Joseph Campbell

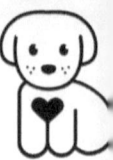

Sticker Square

Date ___ / ___ / ____

Highlights of the past day?

1. _____
2. _____
3. _____

I am grateful for...

1. _____

_____

2. _____

_____

3. _____

_____

I am feeling excited about...

1. _____
2. _____
3. _____

One thing I love about myself is...

_____

"You only live once, but if you do it right, once is enough." ~ Mae West

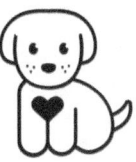

Sticker Square

Date ___ / ___ / ___

Highlights of the past day?

1. _____
2. _____
3. _____

I am grateful for...

1. _____
_____

2. _____
_____

3. _____
_____

I am feeling excited about...

1. _____
2. _____
3. _____

One thing I love about myself is...

_____

"In three words I can sum up everything I've learned about life — It goes on." ~ Robert Frost

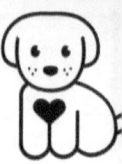

Sticker Square

Date ___ / ___ / ___

Highlights of the past day?

1. _____
2. _____
3. _____

I am grateful for...

1. _____
   _____

2. _____
   _____

3. _____
   _____

I am feeling excited about...

1. _____
2. _____
3. _____

One thing I love about myself is...

_____

"To live is the rarest thing in the world. Most people exist, that is all." ~ Oscar Wilde

Weekly Challenge #27

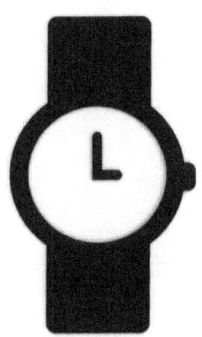

Carpe Diem and refrain from checking the time on your watch/phone/clock this week

Completion Date: __/__/__

Date ___ / ___ / ____

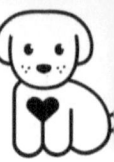

Highlights of the past day?

1. _____
2. _____
3. _____

I am grateful for...

1. _____

_____

2. _____

_____

3. _____

_____

I am feeling excited about...

1. _____
2. _____
3. _____

One thing I love about myself is...

_____

"What counts is not necessarily the size of the dog in the fight—it's the size of the fight in the dog." ~ Dwight Eisenhower

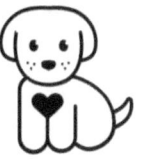

Sticker
Square

Date ___ / ___ / ____

Highlights of the past day?

1. _____
2. _____
3. _____

I am grateful for...

1. _____
   _____

2. _____
   _____

3. _____
   _____

I am feeling excited about...

1. _____
2. _____
3. _____

One thing I love about myself is...

_____

"Don't look for big things, just do small things with great love." ~
Mother Teresa

Date ___ / ___ / ____

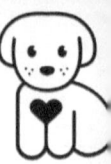

Highlights of the past day?

1. _____
2. _____
3. _____

I am grateful for...

1. _____
_____

2. _____
_____

3. _____
_____

I am feeling excited about...

1. _____
2. _____
3. _____

One thing I love about myself is...

_____

"Fairy tales are more than true—not because they tell us dragons
exist, but because they tell us dragons can be beaten." ~ Neil
Gaiman

Date ___ / ___ / ____

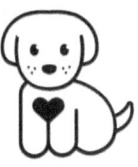

Highlights of the past day?

1. _____
2. _____
3. _____

I am grateful for...

1. _____

_____

2. _____

_____

3. _____

_____

I am feeling excited about...

1. _____
2. _____
3. _____

One thing I love about myself is...

_____

"Love all, trust a few, do wrong to none." ~ Shakespeare

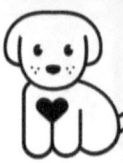

Sticker Square

Date ___ / ___ / ___

Highlights of the past day?

1. _____
2. _____
3. _____

I am grateful for...

1. _____
   _____

2. _____
   _____

3. _____
   _____

I am feeling excited about...

1. _____
2. _____
3. _____

One thing I love about myself is...

_____

"It is our choices . . . that show what we truly are, far more than our abilities." ~ JK Rowling

Weekly Challenge #28

Put your phone on "Do Not Disturb" this week - notice how you feel!

Completion Date: __/__/__

Date ___ / ___ / ___

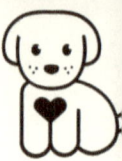

Highlights of the past day?

1. _____
2. _____
3. _____

I am grateful for...

1. _____

   _____

2. _____

   _____

3. _____

   _____

I am feeling excited about...

1. _____
2. _____
3. _____

One thing I love about myself is...

_____

"Unless we stand for something, we shall fall for anything." ~ Peter
Marshall

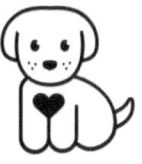
Highlights of the past day?

1. _____
2. _____
3. _____

I am grateful for...

1. _____
   _____

2. _____
   _____

3. _____
   _____

I am feeling excited about...

1. _____
2. _____
3. _____

One thing I love about myself is...

_____

"Be yourself; everyone else is already taken." ~ Oscar Wilde

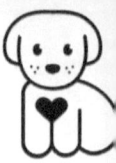

Sticker Square

Date ___ / ___ / ____

Highlights of the past day?

1. _____
2. _____
3. _____

I am grateful for...

1. _____
_____

2. _____
_____

3. _____
_____

I am feeling excited about...

1. _____
2. _____
3. _____

One thing I love about myself is...

_____

"You've gotta' dance like there's nobody watching, Love like you'll never be hurt, Sing like there's nobody listening, And live like it's heaven on earth." ~ William Purkey

Sticker
Square

Date ____ / ____ / ____

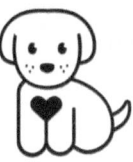

Highlights of the past day?

1. _____
2. _____
3. _____

I am grateful for...

1. _____
   _____

2. _____
   _____

3. _____
   _____

I am feeling excited about...

1. _____
2. _____
3. _____

One thing I love about myself is...

_____

"To be yourself in a world that is constantly trying to make you
something else is the greatest accomplishment." ~ Ralph Waldo
Emerson

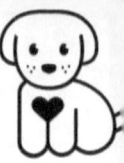

Highlights of the past day?

1. _____
2. _____
3. _____

I am grateful for...

1. _____

_____

2. _____

_____

3. _____

_____

I am feeling excited about...

1. _____
2. _____
3. _____

One thing I love about myself is...

_____

"Always forgive your enemies; nothing annoys them so much." ~
Oscar Wilde

Weekly Challenge #29

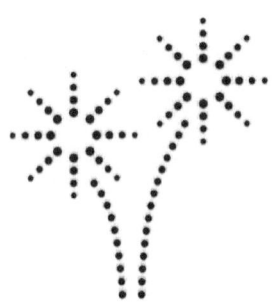

Spend quality time with
one of your parents

My _____ and I _____

Completion Date: __/__/__

Date ___ / ___ / ____

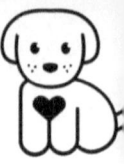

Highlights of the past day?

1. _____
2. _____
3. _____

I am grateful for...

1. _____
_____

2. _____
_____

3. _____
_____

I am feeling excited about...

1. _____
2. _____
3. _____

One thing I love about myself is...

_____

"No one has ever become poor by giving." ~ Anne Frank

Date ___ / ___ / ____

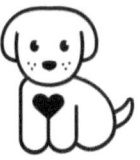

Highlights of the past day?

1. _____
2. _____
3. _____

I am grateful for...

1. _____

_____

2. _____

_____

3. _____

_____

I am feeling excited about...

1. _____
2. _____
3. _____

One thing I love about myself is...

_____

"Don't walk in front of me, I may not follow. Don't walk behind me, I may not lead. Just walk beside me and be my friend." ~ Anon

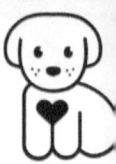

Sticker Square

Date ___ / ___ / ___

Highlights of the past day?

1. _____
2. _____
3. _____

I am grateful for...

1. _____
_____

2. _____
_____

3. _____
_____

I am feeling excited about...

1. _____
2. _____
3. _____

One thing I love about myself is...

_____

"It is never too late to be what you might have been." ~ George Eliot

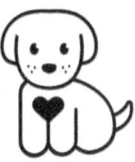

Sticker Square

Date ___ / ___ / ___

Highlights of the past day?

1. _____
2. _____
3. _____

I am grateful for...

1. _____
_____

2. _____
_____

3. _____
_____

I am feeling excited about...

1. _____
2. _____
3. _____

One thing I love about myself is...

_____

"A habit cannot be tossed out the window; it must be coaxed down
the stairs a step at a time." ~ Mark Twain

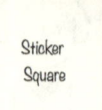

Sticker Square

Date ___ / ___ / ____

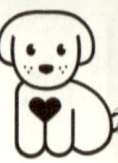

Highlights of the past day?

1. _____
2. _____
3. _____

I am grateful for...

1. _____

_____

2. _____

_____

3. _____

_____

I am feeling excited about...

1. _____
2. _____
3. _____

One thing I love about myself is...

_____

"Life is the flower for which love is the honey." ~ Victor Hugo

Weekly Challenge #30

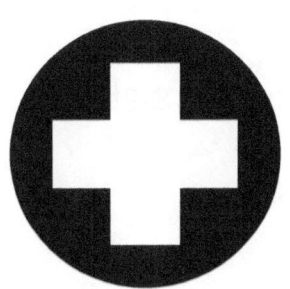

Show some love to a local charity and volunteer their with family/friends.

I volunteered at _____

Completion Date: __/__/__

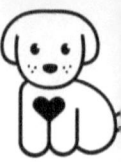

Highlights of the past day?

1. _____
2. _____
3. _____

I am grateful for...

1. _____

_____

2. _____

_____

3. _____

_____

I am feeling excited about...

1. _____
2. _____
3. _____

One thing I love about myself is...

_____

"There are two primary choices in life: to accept conditions as they exist, or accept the responsibility for changing them." ~ Dennis Waitley

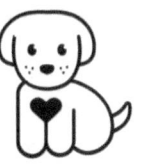

Sticker Square

Date ___ / ___ / ___

Highlights of the past day?

1. _____
2. _____
3. _____

I am grateful for...

1. _____
_____

2. _____
_____

3. _____
_____

I am feeling excited about...

1. _____
2. _____
3. _____

One thing I love about myself is...

_____

"The only thing worse than being blind is having sight but no vision." ~ Helen Keller

Date ___ / ___ / ____

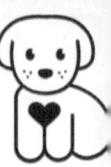

Highlights of the past day?

1. _____
2. _____
3. _____

I am grateful for...

1. _____
_____

2. _____
_____

3. _____
_____

I am feeling excited about...

1. _____
2. _____
3. _____

One thing I love about myself is...

_____

"Remember that happiness is a way of travel, not a destination." ~ Roy Goodman

Date ___ / ___ / ____

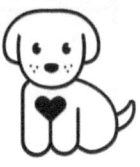

Highlights of the past day?

I. _____
2. _____
3. _____

I am grateful for...

I. _____

_____

2. _____

_____

3. _____

_____

I am feeling excited about...

I. _____
2. _____
3. _____

One thing I love about myself is...

_____

"If not us, who? If not now, when?" ~ Hillel the Elder

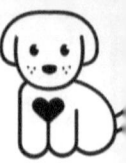

Sticker
Square

Date ___ / ___ / ____

Highlights of the past day?

1. _____
2. _____
3. _____

I am grateful for...

1. _____

_____

2. _____

_____

3. _____

_____

I am feeling excited about...

1. _____
2. _____
3. _____

One thing I love about myself is...

_____

"The best way to predict the future is to invent it." ~ Alan Kay

Weekly Challenge #32

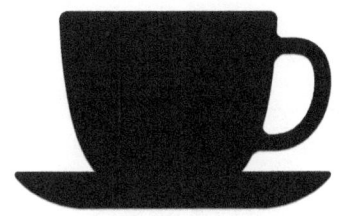

Go to a local coffee shop and treat the barista to their favorite drink. :)

Completion Date: __/__/__

Date ___ / ___ / ___

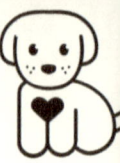

Highlights of the past day?

1. _____
2. _____
3. _____

I am grateful for...

1. _____

_____

2. _____

_____

3. _____

_____

I am feeling excited about...

1. _____
2. _____
3. _____

One thing I love about myself is...

_____

"Failure is the condiment that gives success its flavor." ~ Truman
Capote

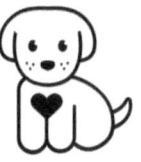

Sticker Square

Date ___ / ___ / ____

Highlights of the past day?

1. _____
2. _____
3. _____

I am grateful for...

1. _____

   _____

2. _____

   _____

3. _____

   _____

I am feeling excited about...

1. _____
2. _____
3. _____

One thing I love about myself is...

_____

"I am only one; but still I am one. I cannot do everything; but still I can do something; and because I cannot do everything, I will not refuse to do the something that I can do" ~Edward Hale

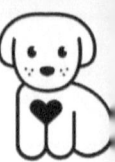

Sticker Square

Date ___ / ___ / ____

Highlights of the past day?

1. _____
2. _____
3. _____

I am grateful for...

1. _____
_____

2. _____
_____

3. _____
_____

I am feeling excited about...

1. _____
2. _____
3. _____

One thing I love about myself is...

_____

"It is not fair to ask of others what you are unwilling to do yourself."
~ Eleanor Roosevelt

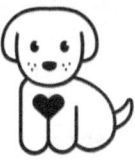

Highlights of the past day?

1. _____
2. _____
3. _____

I am grateful for...

1. _____
_____

2. _____
_____

3. _____
_____

I am feeling excited about...

1. _____
2. _____
3. _____

One thing I love about myself is...

_____

"The elevator to success is out of order. You'll have to use the stairs .
. . one step at a time." ~ Joe Girard

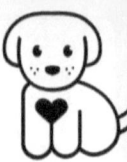

Highlights of the past day?

1. _____
2. _____
3. _____

I am grateful for...

1. _____

    _____

2. _____

    _____

3. _____

    _____

I am feeling excited about...

1. _____
2. _____
3. _____

One thing I love about myself is...

_____

"Life shrinks or expands in proportion to one's courage." ~ Anais Nin

Weekly Challenge #33

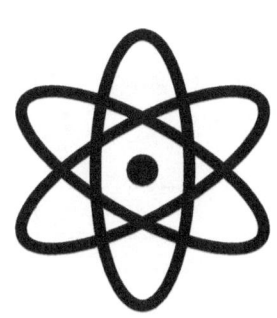

Build an egg parachute and see how well it works!

Completion Date: __/__/__

Date ___ / ___ / ___

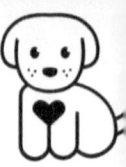

Highlights of the past day?

1. _____
2. _____
3. _____

I am grateful for...

1. _____

_____

2. _____

_____

3. _____

_____

I am feeling excited about...

1. _____
2. _____
3. _____

One thing I love about myself is...

_____

"To the world you may be just one person, but to one person you
may be the world." ~ Brandi Synder

Date ___ / ___ / ____

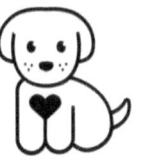

Highlights of the past day?

1. _____
2. _____
3. _____

I am grateful for...

1. _____

   _____

2. _____

   _____

3. _____

   _____

I am feeling excited about...

1. _____
2. _____
3. _____

One thing I love about myself is...

_____

"The conductor of an orchestra doesn't make a sound. He depends,
for his power, on his ability to make other people powerful." ~
Benjamin Zander

Date ___ / ___ / ___

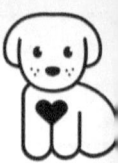

Highlights of the past day?

1. _____
2. _____
3. _____

I am grateful for...

1. _____

   _____

2. _____

   _____

3. _____

   _____

I am feeling excited about...

1. _____
2. _____
3. _____

One thing I love about myself is...

_____

"You see things; and you say "Why?" But I dream things that never
were; and I say "Why not?" " ~ George Bernard Shaw

Sticker
Square

Date ___ / ___ / ____

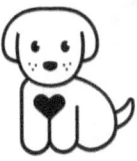

Highlights of the past day?

1. _____
2. _____
3. _____

I am grateful for...

1. _____

_____

2. _____

_____

3. _____

_____

I am feeling excited about...

1. _____
2. _____
3. _____

One thing I love about myself is...

_____

"How wonderful it is that nobody need wait a single moment before
beginning to improve the world." ~ Anne Frank

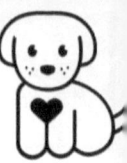

Highlights of the past day?

1. _____
2. _____
3. _____

I am grateful for...

1. _____

_____

2. _____

_____

3. _____

_____

I am feeling excited about...

1. _____
2. _____
3. _____

One thing I love about myself is...

_____

"What lies behind us and what lies before us are tiny matters
compared to what lies within us." ~ Henry Haskins

Weekly Challenge #34

Show a little appreciation to the fam and thank your parents for all they have done for you.

Completion Date: __/__/__

Date ___ / ___ / ___

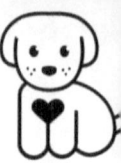

Highlights of the past day?

1. _____
2. _____
3. _____

I am grateful for...

1. _____

_____

2. _____

_____

3. _____

_____

I am feeling excited about...

1. _____
2. _____
3. _____

One thing I love about myself is...

_____

"Not everything that can be counted counts, and not everything
that counts can be counted." ~ William Cameron

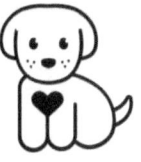

Highlights of the past day?

1. _____
2. _____
3. _____

I am grateful for...

1. _____

_____

2. _____

_____

3. _____

_____

I am feeling excited about...

1. _____
2. _____
3. _____

One thing I love about myself is...

_____

"Courage is contagious. When a brave man takes a stand, the spines of others are stiffened." ~ Billy Graham

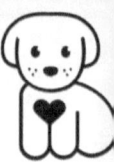

Highlights of the past day?

1. _____
2. _____
3. _____

I am grateful for...

1. _____
_____

2. _____
_____

3. _____
_____

I am feeling excited about...

1. _____
2. _____
3. _____

One thing I love about myself is...

_____

"As a well-spent day brings happy sleep, so a life well spent brings
happy death." ~Leonardo Da Vinci

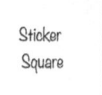

Sticker
Square

Date ___ / ___ / ____

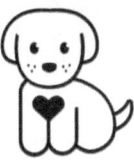

Highlights of the past day?

1. _____
2. _____
3. _____

I am grateful for...

1. _____
_____

2. _____
_____

3. _____
_____

I am feeling excited about...

1. _____
2. _____
3. _____

One thing I love about myself is...

_____

:"All our dreams can come true, if we have the courage to pursue
them." ~ Walt Disney

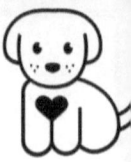

Highlights of the past day?

1. _____
2. _____
3. _____

I am grateful for...

1. _____

_____

2. _____

_____

3. _____

_____

I am feeling excited about...

1. _____
2. _____
3. _____

One thing I love about myself is...

_____

"Wise men speak because they have something to say; fools
because they have to say something." ~ Plato

Weekly Challenge #35

Forgive someone that has hurt you and reach out to them.

I reached out to _____

Completion Date: __/__/__

Sticker Square

Date ___ / ___ / ___

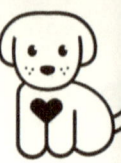

Highlights of the past day?

1. _____
2. _____
3. _____

I am grateful for...

1. _____
_____

2. _____
_____

3. _____
_____

I am feeling excited about...

1. _____
2. _____
3. _____

One thing I love about myself is...

_____

"Just taught my kids about taxes by eating 38% of their ice cream."
~ Conan O'Brien

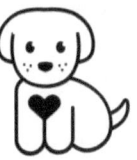

Sticker Square

Date ___ / ___ / ____

Highlights of the past day?

1. _____
2. _____
3. _____

I am grateful for...

1. _____

   _____

2. _____

   _____

3. _____

   _____

I am feeling excited about...

1. _____
2. _____
3. _____

One thing I love about myself is...

_____

"The world is my country, all mankind are my brethren and to do good is my religion." ~ Thomas Paine

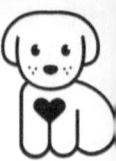

┌─────────┐
│ Sticker │
│ Square │
└─────────┘

Date ___ / ___ / ____

Highlights of the past day?

1. _____
2. _____
3. _____

I am grateful for...

1. _____
   _____

2. _____
   _____

3. _____
   _____

I am feeling excited about...

1. _____
2. _____
3. _____

One thing I love about myself is...

_____

"Worry is like a rocking chair, it will give you something to do, but it
won't get you anywhere." ~ Vance Havner

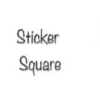
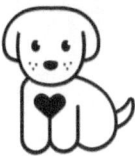
Date ___ / ___ / ____

Highlights of the past day?

1. _____
2. _____
3. _____

I am grateful for...

1. _____

   _____

2. _____

   _____

3. _____

   _____

I am feeling excited about...

1. _____
2. _____
3. _____

One thing I love about myself is...

_____

"I believe in the sacredness of a promise, that a man's word should
be as good as his bond; that character — not wealth or power or
position — is of supreme worth." ~ John Rockefeller

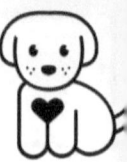

Sticker Square

Date ___ / ___ / ____

Highlights of the past day?

1. _____
2. _____
3. _____

I am grateful for...

1. _____
   _____

2. _____
   _____

3. _____
   _____

I am feeling excited about...

1. _____
2. _____
3. _____

One thing I love about myself is...

_____

"If opportunity doesn't knock, build a door." ~ Milton Berle

Weekly Challenge #36

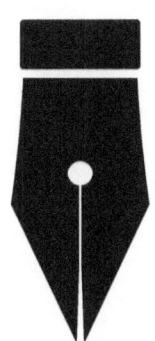

To write or not to write a poem to a friend. May the odds be ever in your favor!

I wrote a poem for _____

Completion Date: __/__/__

Sticker
Square

Date ___ / ___ / ____

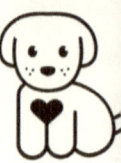

Highlights of the past day?

1. _____
2. _____
3. _____

I am grateful for...

1. _____

   _____

2. _____

   _____

3. _____

   _____

I am feeling excited about...

1. _____
2. _____
3. _____

One thing I love about myself is...

_____

"The next time you're faced with something that's unexpected,
unwanted and uncertain, consider that it just may be a gift." ~
Stacey Kramer

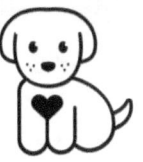

Sticker Square

Date ___ / ___ / ____

Highlights of the past day?

1. _____
2. _____
3. _____

I am grateful for...

1. _____

_____

2. _____

_____

3. _____

_____

I am feeling excited about...

1. _____
2. _____
3. _____

One thing I love about myself is...

_____

"People are illogical, unreasonable, and self-centered. Love them
anyway." ~ Kent Keith

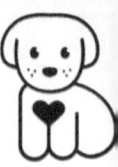

Sticker Square

Date ___ / ___ / ____

Highlights of the past day?

1. _____
2. _____
3. _____

I am grateful for...

1. _____

_____

2. _____

_____

3. _____

_____

I am feeling excited about...

1. _____
2. _____
3. _____

One thing I love about myself is...

_____

"Never doubt that a small group of thoughtful, committed citizens can change the world. Indeed, it's the only thing that ever has." ~ Margaret Mead

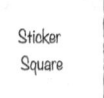

Sticker
Square

Date ___ / ___ / ____

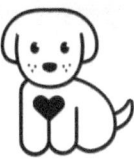

Highlights of the past day?

1. _____
2. _____
3. _____

I am grateful for...

1. _____
   _____

2. _____
   _____

3. _____
   _____

I am feeling excited about...

1. _____
2. _____
3. _____

One thing I love about myself is...

_____

"Either you run the day, or the day runs you." ~ Jim Rohn

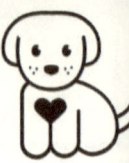

Date ___ / ___ / ____

Highlights of the past day?

1. _____
2. _____
3. _____

I am grateful for...

1. _____

_____

2. _____

_____

3. _____

_____

I am feeling excited about...

1. _____
2. _____
3. _____

One thing I love about myself is...

_____

"Don't cry because it's over, smile because it happened." ~ Theodor
Geisel

Final Challenge

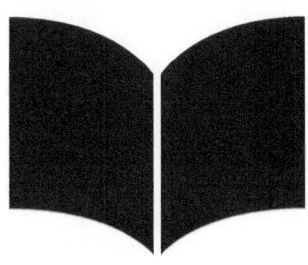

Look back through this journal and reflect on your gratitude journey!

_____
_____
_____
_____
_____
_____
_____
_____
_____
_____